Johnny Rocke

Summary of:

The Obesity Code & the Diabetes Code by Dr. Jason Fung. Unlocking the Secrets of Weight Loss

---

Prevent and Reverse Type 2 Diabetes Naturally

Revised Transcripts

25% of the royalties will go to Dr. Fung's research and work via donation!

P.S.: Any review would be GREATLY appreciated to get the Low-Carb message out!

TABLE OF CONTENTS

Chapter 1

Jason Fung - Solving the two compartment problem

So what we're going to talk about today is really why intermittent fasting and low carbohydrate diets work whereas the calorie counters, it just doesn't seem to work. Right? And the problem with the calorie theory is that it's just like, wrong. And, because we don't really understand obesity, that's why we can't cure it. Right?

I'm sure many of you have seen this show, it's called "The Biggest Loser" and it's on North America, it's in Australia, it's everywhere right? Now, what people do is they're contestants that compete to lose weight and they get put on a diet. It's a calorie reduced diet and they did do a lot of exercise and you've seen Jillian Michaels screaming at everybody, right? So it's a lot of exercise and... they don't show it on the show but there's actually a fairly severe caloric restriction as well. It's not a low carbohydrate diet, its more of a 'everything in moderation' approach.

So the problem, of course, is that... this show has been running for a long time and certain of the contestants have come out and said, "Well, you know this really doesn't work!" Now, the reason more haven't come out is because they're essentially under a legal gag order, right? They're actually not allowed to say any of this stuff:

The Biggest Loser

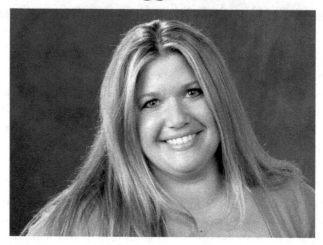

„NBC never does a reunion. Why? We're all fat again"
Susanne Mendonca – Season 2

But certain contestants have actually come out and so this contestant Susan said, "Well, they never do a reunion show. Why? They've all gained that weight again."

And it's not unique to "The Biggest Loser", we've all done these calorie reduced diets, it does the same for everybody. It does fine for about six months - but then after that it just keeps coming back. Your weight plateaus, then it starts to come back! And everybody knows this, right, because everybody's done this diet. The question is why? And that's what we really have to understand and that's what I mean by we have to solve the two compartment problem.

So *The Biggest Loser-* diet, despite the fact that we all know it doesn't work, is actually ranked very highly. So USA News, for example, just this past year put The Biggest Loser diet at number three for weight loss and number eleven overall:

The Biggest Loser Diet

- Reduce Calories

- Increase Exercise

- Eat Less, Move More!

- 2015 Rankings

    - #3 Weight Loss

    - #11 Overall

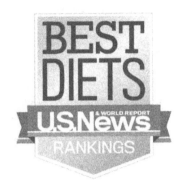

Where's the evidence that reducing calories causes weight loss?

So really a very good diet then. Why not? It's a *eat less, move more* sort of approach. Right? Cut your calories in, increase your calories out, and hey, presto, you're gonna lose weight. So that's why it does so well, all the doctors recommend it and so on.

The thing is that there have been some studies, that have been done on these contestants. And it's very interesting to look scientifically at what actually happens to these people as they do this eat less, move more approach. Now, The Biggest Loser of course is that approach on steroids, right? So you're eating a lot less and you're moving a lot more and that's why you get these dramatic weight losses.

So one season, they actually took these contestants, made them sign consent and then actually did metabolic studies on them. And what's interesting is that: At first it looks amazing, right, and we've all seen that show, the befores and the afters - looks amazing! And the studies really bear that out.

So if you look at the before and after, if you look at the composition of weight loss so at week six and week thirty (and the end of the show is week thirty) you can see that they lost a lot of weight. Right? This is sixty kilograms:

The Biggest Loser

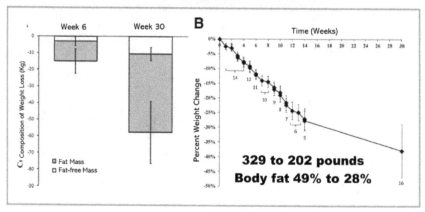

Metabolic slowing with massive weight loss despite preservation of fat-free mass.
Johannsen DL et al., J Clin Endocrinol Metab., 2012; 97(7); 2489-96

And this is fat mass. Most of it is fat. Right? Everybody says, "Ah you're gonna lose muscle, you're gonna lose muscle". Their losing mostly fat, there's a little bit of muscle loss but it's mostly fat.

And this is their body fat percentage and you can see, it follows a pretty steady trend downwards. The average participant went from 329nine pounds to 202 pounds so amazing results, right? Body fat went from 49 percent to 28 percent.

So at the end of the show you get these great results, you have the end of the show, everybody wins and they pretend like everything's fine. But we know that it isn't.

And why not? What's the problem? It sounds like it should work, right? You keep doing what you're doing and you'll keep losing weight. But you don't. And the reason - and we've known this for at least a hundred years - is that your metabolism starts to slow down. And this is what happened to the metabolism of all these contestants:

Decreased Metabolism

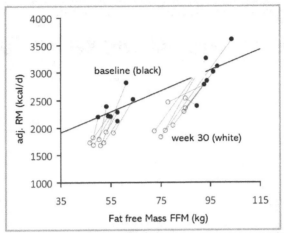

Metabolic slowing with massive weight loss despite preservation of fat-free mass.
Johannsen DL et al., J Clin Endocrinol Metab., 2012; 97(7); 2489-96

And you can see in the black circles above the solid bar (that's their baseline rate of metabolism before they started this) and the open circles is that afterwards. You can see that in virtually every case these people are cutting the amount of calories they expend by a lot, okay?

So you can look at some of these dramatic examples. One fellow for example is starts out by burning 3500 calories a day and he's dropped all the way to about 1700 calories a day! And it's not just him, it's everybody. If you take the entire group of people, the average decrease in metabolism is over 700 calories a day. Right? So you start at two thousand you're gonna drop down to like 1200, 1300 by the end of the show.

So you wonder why you're not losing weight. Well, it's because your metabolism has slowed down so much that if you're burning 1300 and you are eating 1500 (remember that's still a lot less than you used to eat) you're gonna gain the weight back. That's exactly what we all know happens. You feel cold, you feel tired, you feel hungry, you feel like shit - and the weight is going back up! Right? And that's the problem.

We all know that's the problem. It's the decrease in metabolism. So you can try to make up for it with more exercise. And that's what they pretend that you can do.

Decreased Metabolism

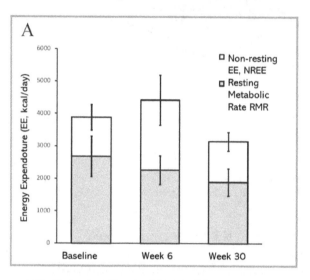

J Clin Endocrinol Metab., 2012; 97(7); 2489-96

So you can see at baseline, there's a certain amount which is resting metabolic rate, certain amount of exercise. During the show they burn a hell of a lot of calories as exercise. You see that they've ramped up, so your total energy expenditure is better.

But, when you stop exercising for like, you know, five hours a day, then your exercise goes down... but look at what happened to your basal metabolism. This is your resting metabolic rate. It's already gone down by week six, okay? So don't kid yourself – this is happening all the time. But by week thirty, it's gone down even more. And that's the whole problem, you get this metabolic slowdown.

And because you're not burning as much energy you don't have that liveliness. You don't feel very good. And you can see this in the graph above, you see the "The Biggest Loser" contestants, and you see that the basal metabolic rate just keeps on going down.

But there's a similar extreme measure that doesn't seem to have this problem and the question is why. So you can look at Bariatric surgery, Bariatric surgery is stomach stapling surgery. So you cut your stomach into the size of a walnut, you really just can't eat. And you can't eat for months and months and months, and guess what? The weight goes down, right?

That's not a surprise. The surprise is that it works to keep weight off in the long term. Yeah, there are a lot of problems with this, okay? Let's be clear I'm not recommending it for anybody. But if you look at the resting metabolic rate with a similarly, sort of, extreme measure it goes back up.

Biggest Loser vs. Bariatrics

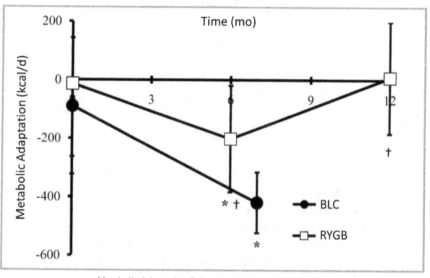

Metabolic Adaptation Following Massive Weight Loss (..)
Knuth ND et al, Obesity 2014; 22: 2563-2569

The question is why?
This is another study of the long-term effects of Bariatrics:

Long Term Effect of Bariatrics

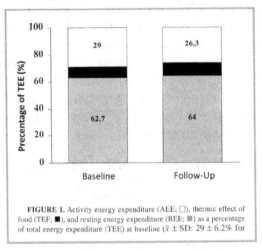

FIGURE 1. Activity energy expenditure (AEE; ▫), thermic effect of food (TEF; ■), and resting energy expenditure (REE; ▥) as a percentage of total energy expenditure (TEE) at baseline (x̄ ± SD: 29 ± 6.2% for

Long-term changes in energy expenditure and body composition after massive weight loss (...)
Krupa Das S et al, Am J Clin Nu 2003 78: 22-30

You can see that at baseline and at follow-up (this is several years later) the resting metabolic rate and the total energy expenditure (how much energy or burning) has really not gone down. As opposed to the eat less, move more, where it keeps going down, keeps going down until you fail. Right?

That of course is the saddest part of all. The saddest part of the entire thing is that we know about this metabolic slowdown. This was shown in 1915, so we've known about it for a hundred years.

What I think is sad is that we give people this really horrific advice to eat less and move more... and then when they fail we blame them for it. That's basically blaming the victim. Because, here's this poor fellow or poor lady who's victimized because they're suffering from obesity, from type 2 diabetes. You give them really bad advice which you know is gonna fail - because we've all done it fails, every single time - and then, when the weight goes back you say, "Yeah you should have listened to me better, you should have more willpower, you shouldn't have eaten that bagel" or whatever it is you tell people.

And that's really the saddest part of all, is that we try to pretend that the advice that we give is really good and the failure lies with all of you. Right? That doesn't doesn't make any sense. How can 40, 50 percent of the population be so morally bankrupt that they let this happen to them? Is it not more logical that the advice that we gave was just really crappy? That seems to me much more sensible.

So we're gonna explain why this sort of discrepancy exists. In order to do that you have to understand what happens when you eat. Okay? So what happens when you eat is that insulin goes up. So most foods, almost all foods, have a mixture of macro-nutrients,: Fats, carbohydrates and protein. So your insulin goes up to a varying degree:

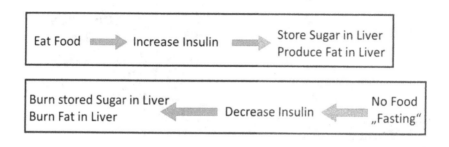

Storage:

Glycogen (sugar)   Fridge
Fat   Freezer

And insulin basically is the hormone that tells your body to store fat, so it stops your body from burning fat, you start to store some of the sugar and youstore some of the fat. Okay? And this is normal, this is a normal situation.

Carbohydrates get turned into glycogen which are chains of glucose, the chains of glucose in the liver is basically a storage form of sugar. And when you have too much of that, then your liver produces lipids - which is called "de novo lipogenesis" - and it basically stores fat. Okay?

So when you don't eat (when you're fasting, so fasting is merely the absence of eating) your insulin levels fall. And that's a signal to start pulling some of that energy out. So you're gonna start by pulling some energy out from the glycogen which is your stored sugar, and you're going to pull some energy out of the stored fat.

So you can think of the glycogen like a refrigerator. You're storing food energy. And the reason it's like a refrigerator is that it's easy to access. So you can put food in easily, you can take food out easily. Right? It's just food energy.

Two Compartment Model

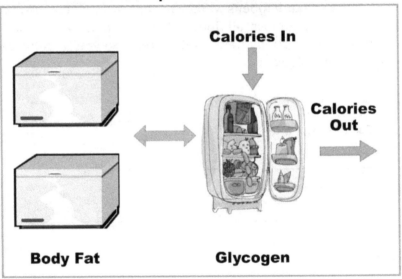

And the fat is more like your freezer. Okay? So you can store more of it, but it's in your basement, you know, it's hard to get to, it's hard to get out, it's hard to put in. So you generally prefer to use your refrigerator. And it's the same idea, you have two storage forms of energy. One easy to use, then one not so easy to use. The refrigerator though has a limited capacity, so if you have too much stuff you have no choice but to put it in your freezer.

Now, the reason that the calories don't work is that they operate on what I call a "one compartment model." That means, they pretend, that all your calories that go in to your body are all the same. All your calories are the same, they're stored in one giant compartment (like this sink) and when it comes to taking out energy it all comes out of the same thing:

One Compartment Model

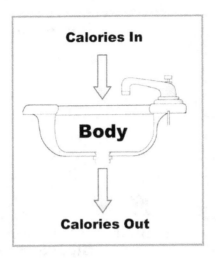

Right? Therefore, if you follow this very simplistic incorrect model, what you see is that if you'd simply reduce the calories going in, you'll reduce your weight. And if you increase the calories out, you'll increase the rate. But this entire premise of this *calories in, calories out model* is completely fictitious because we know that's not what happens in the body!

The body doesn't have some giant vat of calories. Right? You can store sugar, you can store fat. It's not some giant vat of calories that's held somewherei in your liver. Right? But that's what they all pretend it is. So if you have the entire wrong idea of why this should work, then it's not gonna work.

What instead is a better model, is a two compartment model. That is, there are two places in the body where you can store food.

You've got your fridge and you've got your freezer:

Two Compartment Model

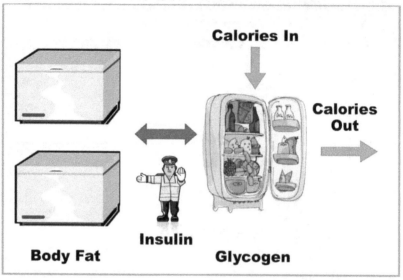

Your calories go in into your fridge and your calories go out from the fridge because that's the easiest place. But there's a third thing that you have to consider and that is how much food goes back and forth between the freezer and the fridge, because that's what we're really interested in: the fat! That's the one that's much harder to get too. Right? And the question is, what's controlling this, because that's really the key.

It turns out that the main player is insulin. We know this because insulin inhibits lipolysis. What that means is it stops you from getting the fat coming out. That's its job, that's its normal job. So if you have a lot of insulin... so normally, if you eat a huge meal your insulin is high, it's gonna tell the body to move all the storage in this way. If your insulin is very high then you can't get the food back out this way. And that's the problem.

If you have a lot of insulin resistance, for example, which keeps your insulin levels very high, it's like that freezer is kind of locked away in the basement behind a locked steel bar. You can't get at it.

So what happens now when you start reducing your calories? If you start reducing your calories in and you can't get at your storage, what your body is simply gonna do is reduce the calories out. That's what it does.Right? Because it's not gonna keep losing weight until you die, that's just ridiculous.

If you look at the *Women's Health Initiative* (which was a huge 50,000 person study) they reduced calories by 350 per day, for seven years. And they estimated that people would lose thirty pounds. Women would lose thirty pounds per year. Right? So in seven years they should have lost two hundred and ten pounds. Right?

Of course, that didn't happen. How much did they lose? Not even a single pound. It was ridiculous! Because what happened, of course, was that their body... if you're not affecting the insulin, you can't get at that fat. You're just going to reduce your calories out.

And notice here, of course, that we're not breaking any laws of thermodynamics. Right? Calories in, calories out. Yeah, your accounting for all the calories but what's important is the compartmentalization of energy. That's what we're talking about, not the total energy, but where it goes.

Because that's what we want to know. If you eat and you just burn it off - who cares? That'd be great! But if you eat and all of it goes into fat, well, now you care a lot. Right? But it's not that calories are in balance, if you eat an extra five hundred calories your body burns it all off as heat, who cares? You don't have any extra body fat. But if you eat five hundred extra calories, the insulin is telling it all to shove int the freezer, well that's a problem. And that's really the problem of the two compartment syndrome.

So if you look at what happens during fasting... what happens? Because everybody worries about this, right? "Oh, what about protein? You're burning your muscles!" This is a study by Kevin Hall from the NIH and he basically looked what happens during fasting. This is what happens:

Fuel usage during Fasting

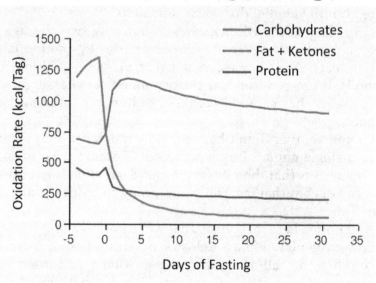

Comparative Physiology of Fasting, Starvation and Food Limitation, Autor: Dr. Kevin Hall, NIH

So for the first couple of days of fasting, what you see is that carbohydrate oxidation goes up, it goes way up. In other words you're burning sugar. You can see that fat doesn't actually move for a couple of days. You're not burning a hell of a lot of fat. And then, as you run out of the glycogen... remember that the glycogen is your easily accessed energy but limited in terms of how much you can store. Once it all burns out, then look: fat oxidation goes up. Now you're burning fat for energy. That's perfect. That's exactly what we want to do.

What happened to protein? Are you burning muscle? Hell no! It goes up slightly, okay, at the very beginning, then drops. Protein is not a storage form of energy. Why would your body burn it for energy? You hear this argument all the time, "You're gonna burn muscle!" Right? So it's ridiculous because you are telling me that the way we are designed is to store energy as fat, but when the chips are down we'll burn muscle? Okay, like I don't think so. Crazy!

It's like if you have a wood-burning stove, you store firewood because you're gonna burn it. But when the chips are down you don't go chop up your sofa and throw it into the fire. Right? It's crazy!

The other thing that's ridiculous is that if you have repeated fast-famine cycles, like cavemen might have had for instance... you store fat, burn muscle. So at the end of a few of these cycles you're like one giant ball of hundred percent fat, right? It's like that's what happens to the bears.

It's like, come on, don't be ridiculous, you don't burn muscle. Protein - yes, you do need a certain amount of protein to maintain your lean protein, right, But it's not increased. That's my point. It's not that it's not zero, there is some, right, but it's not increased in response to fasting.

So the reason that I talk about fasting and low-carbohydrate diets is what it does very effectively (and probably more effectively than any other intervention) is it empties out that fridge:

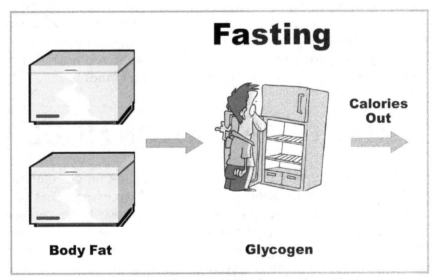

„Medical Bariatrics"

Remember, what you want to do is get rid of all that insulin too. Because now, if you don't have insulin telling your body to shunt all that energy into fat, now you can start to move your calories out this way. If you have a lot of insulin... so we do this, for example, if we give people exogenous insulin they can't lose weight. Right? Even if they fast it was very hard because they can't access that fat. They just keep reducing their calorie expenditure. But the whole point is that fasting provides the easiest way to get rid of all that glycogen, you get your insulin down so you can actually access your body fat!

And the whole thing is that why can't you fast? I asked my son one time a few years ago, you know, "How do you lose weight?" He goes (he was six or seven at the time) "Just don't eat!". So easy, right? It's like, "Huh, how can you be so right about this point that has escaped like 99% of the worlds doctors and dietitians?" Right? If you don't eat you're gonna lose weight and here's the thing to understand: there's nothing wrong with it!

That's the way we're built. That's the way lions are built, thats the way tigers are built, thats the way bears are built, that's the way we're built. We're built to withstand these repeated episodes where there's no food. Right? Because back in the caveman days there's no McDonald's, there's no refrigerator, there's nothing. There are times when you're gonna have nothing, that's why you have fat. Right? That's the whole point.

One of the most ironic things is this is, what you hear all the time, "Fasting is gonna put you into starvation mode".

MYTH - STARVATION MODE

This is actually very ironic because starvation mode refers to the idea that your metabolism slows to such an extent, that you are going to regain weight. Okay? so I've heard that before somewhere. That's exactly what happens when you try to reduce your calories. Right? If you don't do anything about your insulin and just reduce your calories your metabolism goes down. You're going into starvation mode. But what happens during fasting? Does it happen?

Well, here's a study of four consecutive days of fasting:

Metabolic Changes over 4 days of fasting

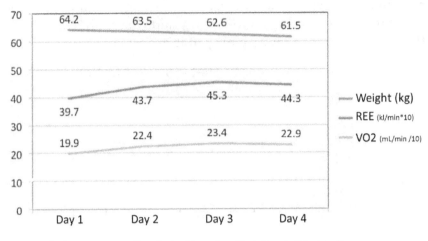

Resting energy expenditure in short-term starvation is increased as a result of an increase in serum norepinephrine.
Zauner C et al, Am J Clin Nutr 2000; 71(6):1511-5

This is a normal people. And what you see is that at the top the weight goes down. So that's great, that's exactly what we expect to see. But what happens to your REE? This is this middle line here. That's the "Resting Energy Expenditure". That's your basal metabolism. It doesn't go down, it goes up! Right? You're burning more energy than you did.

Now you might think why is that so? Well, it makes a lot of sense, because, suppose again you're a caveman and there's nothing to eat. It's winter there's nothing to eat. So if your body starts shutting down, then you're even less likely to find something to eat - 'cause you're tired. You can't go out there and hunt a woolly mammoth, you're tired. Right? You need to sleep. So that's gonna... you're all going to die like that!

Your body is just not that stupid. Your body says, "Well, you have nothing to eat, so I'm gonna give you energy. I'm gonna increase the amount of energy you're burning and I'm gonna provide it from your fat stores, because you need to go out and eat and fill up this refrigerator again." So that's exactly what you do, otherwise we wouldn't be here. It'd be like cockroaches and insects were running the world.

So what happens to your VO2? That's how much oxygen you can metabolize. Does it slow down? No, it goes up! Again, you have more capacity to do exercise, more energy - and why is that so? One, you're burning fat for energy and your body's like, "Hoo there's a lot of this, there's plenty of it, let's go!"

Metabolic changes over 4 days of fasting

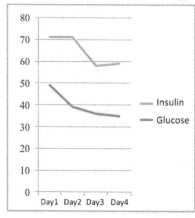 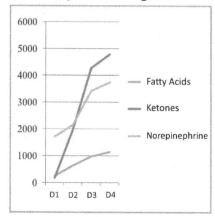

Zauner C et al, Am J Clin Nutr 2000; 71(6):1511-5

But the other thing you see is that the norepinephrine (so norepinephrine and epinephrine are called adrenaline, or noradrenaline) so your body is actually providing you with a big kick in the pants to keep your energy expenditure high - because that's what you need to do to survive! So insulin drops which is one of the major things that we want to see, and your hormones (remember, obesity is a hormonal disease) it goes up. It's providing you the tools to burn fat. So there's no starvation mode, actually its quite the opposite! It goes up.

You can do something called *alternate daily fasting* which is kind of one day of fasting and one off. In these studies it's not actually a full fast they still allowed about 500 calories on those fasting days. So it's not even a true fast. But the calories are low enough that you still get the benefits.

22 Days Alternate Daily Fasting

	Baseline c	Day 21	Day 22
RMR (kJ/d)	6675 ± 283	6292 ± 268	6329 ± 260
RQ	0.85 ± 0.01	0.86 ± 0.02	$0.79 ± 0.01^2$
Fat oxidation (g/24 h)^3	64 ± 8	54 ± 10	$101 ± 9^2$
Carbohydrate oxidation (g/24 h)^3	175 ± 17	184 ± 24	$81 ± 16^2$

RMR = Resting Metabolic Rate

Alternate-day fasting in nonobese subjects: effects on body weight, body composition, and energy metabolism.
Heilbronn LK et al, Am J Clin Nutr 2005; 81:69-73

And again, if you look at their resting metabolic rate you can see that from baseline to day twenty-two (a couple of weeks of alternate daily fasting) your resting metabolic rate really hasn't dropped. Your fat oxidation goes way up. Right? So you're burning fat. You can't argue with that, right? You can measure these things, you're burning fat. Why? Because you have no carbohydrates to burn. Because you're clearing out that fridge, you're clearing out all that stored sugar and burning fat. That's great, that's exactly what we want to do.

MYTH - BURN MUCLE

The other thing we talked a little bit about already is that you're gonna burn muscle. And again, the idea is that you're going to burn protein to provide glucose. Right? And this doesn't actually happen.

This has been known, again, for twenty, twenty-five years:

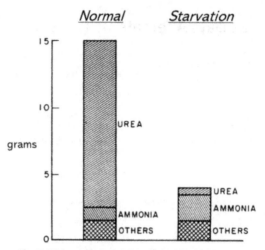

Fig. 5: Nitrogen Excretion (in g/24h) falls during starvation

Starvation – in 'Transaction of the American Clinical and Climatological Association'. Cahill, G. 1983; 02/1983; 94; 1-21

So if you look at Urea, Urea is this big line here. So it's a breakdown product of protein. You can see that you excrete a certain amount of nitrogen everyday. You're also taking in a certain amount of nitrogen everyday. This under normal conditions. Nowyou fast people. You just give them nothing to eat. Well what happens? Well, there's virtually no urea coming out.

There's nothing going in, too. But what you notice is that you're not burning muscle. Because if you're burning muscle that urea should skyrocket or at least be as high as on the left side. But your body is actively conserving your protein, your muscle mass. Right? And that's what happens during fasting.

And you can do 70 days of alternate daily fasting. Seventy days is more than two and a bit months:

Burn Muscle

	Baseline control phase		Weight loss/ADF self-selected feeding phase	
	Day 1	Day 14	Day 69 Feed day	Day 70 Fast day
Body weight (kg)	96.4 ± 5.3	96.5 ± 5.2	92.8 ± 4.8*	90.8 ± 4.8*
BMI (kg/m²)	33.7 ± 1.0	33.7 ± 1.0	32.1 ± 0.8*	31.4 ± 0.9*
Fat mass (kg)	43.0 ± 2.2	43.5 ± 2.5	38.1 ± 2.6*	38.1 ± 1.8*
Fat-free mass (kg)	52.0 ± 3.6	51.4 ± 3.4	52.8 ± 3.3	51.9 ± 3.7
Waist circumference (cm)	109 ± 2	109 ± 3	105 ± 3*	105 ± 3*

Improvements in Coronary Heart Disease Risk Indicators by Alternate-Day Fasting(..)
Bhutani S et al, Obesity (2010) 18, 2152-2159.

And what you see is that if you measure fat mass and fat-free mass in this study, you can see that fat mass goes down very nicely from 43.5 to 38.1 kilos. And the fat-free mass, your lean mass, doesn't move at all.

So, these aresome of the myths that everybody tells you, right? Starvation mode, burning protein and here's my favorite: "It doesn't work, that's never going to work!"

MYTH - IT DOESN'T WORK!

Right? It's like, "Okay genius. If you don't eat, do you think you will lose weight?" Well, yes, you will. So it's not exactly a very good comeback for people to say it won't work, because it will definitely work.

If I don't eat, will I lose weight?

It will definitely work. I'm not saying it's easy, okay? That's a whole other thing. Can you do it? That's a separate question. I actually think that most people can do it. But if you are able to do it, yes, you will lose weight.

And, here's the thing. So, back in the 1960s they have done a bunch of studies on these patients - and they just watched them and you can see that people lose weight:

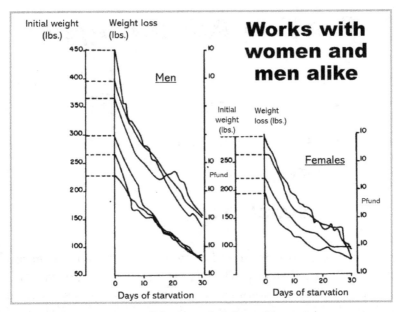

Influence of Fasting and Refeeding on Body Composition.
Drenick EJ et al, Am J Public Health Nations. 1968; 58 (3): 477-484

And here's the thing that is always said. People are going, "How about women? Women shouldn't fast!" Like, why not? Don't you think you'll lose weight? Yes you will. Now, if you're underweight, then yeah, you shouldn't be fasting, right? You're gonna get amenorrhea, you're gonna get menstrual problems, But if you need to lose weight, yes, you will lose weight. And that's exactly what they found in all these studies.

So you have men - they lose weight. Women - they lose weight, too! Right? And what you can see that it's fairly steady, there's no kind of drop off. There's no drop off, that kind of dreaded weight plateau. Because that's the whole problem with weight regain is that we all plateau.

And there's so many advantages to fasting that are just not available in that it's completely different from most other diets which tell you what to do. Beause this is really the opposite, it's something you don't do. Right? So one of the biggest advantages is really that it's completely simple.

Fasting Advantages

- **Flexibility**
- **Convenience**
- **Free**
- **Simplicity**

You can explain it in like two seconds and everybody understands intrinsically what it is. Now, there are variations right? There's fat fast, there's juice fast, there's, you know, water only fast, there's no water fast. There's all kinds of variations but at its very core its easy to understand. And that's important because if people don't understand what you're trying to do, they can't do it.

It's free. Like, you know, as much as I would love to always eat home cooked meals, and, you know, long simmered bone broth, the truth is that most of us sometimes don't have the time and don't have the inclination. Don't have the money... if you want to eat grass fed beef every day, it's gonna cost you. You wanna eat organic all the time, it's going to cost you. I'm not saying that you shouldn't but it's expensive and some people just have no money.

So I have people who write me from the Philippines and they're like "I can't afford anything!" It's like, well, there is no cost, there's no cost at all. It's convenient. Right? So again, you can cookay all you want but it takes time. It takes time, and sometimes you just don't have the time.

But with fasting, there's no shopping, there's no preparation, there's no cooking, there's no clean up, there's no eating. Right? There's nothing. It's so convenient. Beause again, the key is it's not something to -do-, it's something to -not- do. Right?

And that makes it completely different and something that you can add, something that's completely flexible. So it's not like "Oh

26

yeah, you need to eat six times a day!" Sometimes you just don't wanna eat six times a day. Sometimes you're busy, Well, this is gonna give you more time, you can put it in anywhere. You can do it tomorrow and you can not do it the whole next week - and then do it again. Right? You can do whatever you want, it's completely flexible. You can do it for 12 hours, you can do it for 12 days. It doesn't matter.

And really the point is that you can add it to any diet because again it's something that you can put in and fit in wherever you need to:

Add To Any Diet

You don't eat meat?
You don't eat wheat?
You have a nut allergy?
You don't have time?
You don't have money?
You are travelling all the time?
You don't cook?

So say you wanna eat the rice diet or something like that. You can still fast, right? That's the whole point. You don't eat meat? you can still fast. You don't eat wheat, you can still fast. You have a nut allergy, you can still fast. You don't have time, right? Hey, you can still fast. You don't have money, you can still fast. You're traveling all day, you can still fast. You don't cook. Yeah. You can still fast.

And probably the most important thing is that it really has unlimited power:

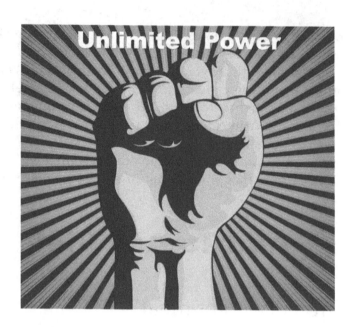

And as a doctor sometimes you get into these things where you want to do something and it's not strong enough. Well, you can just keep fasting until you get the results you want. As I said, if you don't eat you will lose weight. It's almost impossible to not.

Can you keep it up? That's a separate question. I'm not saying it's easy. I'm not saying that you don't have to have the proper medical supervision, especially if you're on medications so on. But you could fast, you could fast. I have a 75 year old who did like thirty days. Right? He felt great. The world record is 382 days. You can keep going.

The whole point is that this gives you options, because it's not a diet. It's no diet, it's nothing. It's like Costanza, "It's a show about nothing!" George Costanza was so smart. That's the whole point is that because it's the opposite it gives you so much flexibility. And it has the ability to really free ourselves of the chains that bind us down. Right?

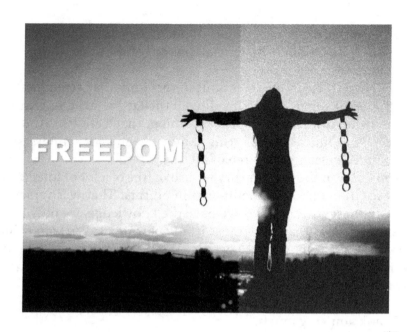

We have all these problems in the world today. You got heart attacks, you got cancer, you got strokes, you got diabetes, you got kidney disease and it's all due to obesity. It's all due to diabetes. But yet, we have the ability to free ourselves from all of these modern afflictions. Only with the application of a technique they knew 5,000 years ago.

The ancient Greeks were all about fasting. Not for health (they didn't have a lot of obesity back then) but because it gave you energy, gave you mental focus. That's why they did it. And these involuntary periods of fasting eventually got taken out as we started getting more reliable food.

Then religion started introducing periods of fasting. So if you look at any major religion in the world, they have periods of fasting. They have periods of feasting, too. But it's balanced by periods of fasting. And remember that they're not trying to kill all their practitioners. They're not like, "Ah, you should fast, ah, you'll die, haha!" That's not it at all. Right?

They did it because there is something deeply, intrinsically beneficial to the fasting. And it was always known, always; It's a cleanse, it's a detox. Right? There's probably only one thing that the three most influential people in the history of the world agreed on. The Prophet Muhammad, Jesus Christ and Buddha.

They all agreed on one thing - and that is fasting. It is very beneficial, its uniquely beneficial, not only for the spirit but also for your body.

We need to clean ourselves out of this junk that accumulates. All this extra sugar, all the insulin, all the fat, we need to clean it out once in awhile. It's a spring cleaning, that's all it is. And yet with the application of this kind of ancient time-tested technique, we can break free of all this.

You know in the last century we broke free of a lot of infectious diseases, tuberculosis, pneumonia in all this. That was replaced with all these diseases. But we have the knowledge, we only have to apply it. And that's the most ironic part of all: We won't. But there's no reason why we won't. We've always been told by everybody that we have to do that this - and yet why do we not? My son knew it.

Thank you very much.

Dr. Jason Fung: A New Paradigm of Insulin Resistance

How to Reverse Type 2 Diabetes Naturally

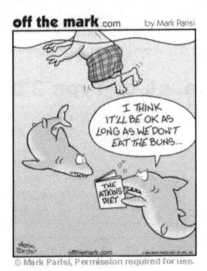

So today what we're going to talk about is insulin resistance because that's really the heart of type 2 diabetes. This is my disclosure:

Presenter Disclosure

- Presenters – Jason Fung

- Relationships with commercial interests:
  - Grants/Research Support: None
  - Grants/Speakers Bureau/Honoria: None
  - Consulting Fees: None
  - Other: None

I don't really have any commercial interest.

Type 2 diabetes is a really important disease because it causes (or is associated with) most of the diseases that we care about today - which is heart disease, cancer, Alzheimer's disease and so on. But we really have to think about this insulin resistance in a new paradigm. Because the one that we've been taught, the one that we understand, actually isn't the one that's really true.

And so type 2 diabetes is a disease with two phases, right? If you look at the time course of the blood glucose before the diagnosis of type 2 diabetes, there's actually two phases:

Two Phases of Type 2 Diabetes

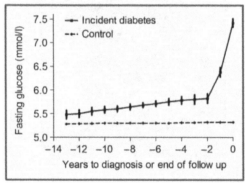

FIGURE 1 Change in fasting plasma glucose during the 13 years prior to onset of Type 2 diabetes. These data from the Whitehall II study demonstrate the elevation of plasma glucose within the normal range

Trajectories of glycaemia, insulin sensitivity, and insulin secretion before diagnosis of type 2 diabetes: an analysis from the Whitehall II study. Lancet 2009; 373: 2215-2221

So there's a long slow phase where the blood glucose rises very, very slowly. That's where the insulin resistance is rising. But the body produces enough insulin to overcome this resistance. So the blood glucose stays relatively normal, it's compensated. Right? So it's called a "compensatory hyperinsulinemia".

At some point the pancreas doesn't produce sufficient insulin. Either the insulin resistance is too high or the amount of insulin drops. So because you lose this compensation, the blood glucose goes up and type 2 diabetes is diagnosed. But that's relatively late in the game.

The image shows you that even up to 14 years prior to the diagnosis of type 2 diabetes, you get this rising insulin resistance:

Insulin Resistance

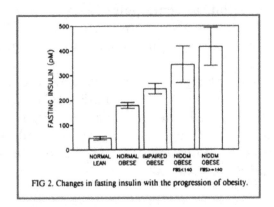

FIG 2. Changes in fasting insulin with the progression of obesity.

Surgical treatment of obesity and ist effect on diabetes: 10-y follow-up
Am J Clin Nutr 1992: 55 (Suppl.): 582S-585S

You can see this when you look across the spectrum of lean people and obese people - as they develop more and more pre-diabetes and diabetes, insulin resistance goes up and up.

This is a slide of the beta cells so the beta cells in the pancreas produce insulin, this is the black circles:

Beta Cell Dysfunction

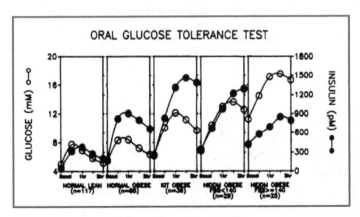

Surgical treatment of obesity and ist effect on diabetes: 10-y follow-up
Am J Clin Nutr 1992: 55 (Suppl.): 582S-585S

You can see as you go across the spectrum from normal to obese to pre-diabetes to diabetes, insulin production initially goes up. So, as you go to the middle - the black circles- you can see that it goes up but at some point it drops. And the white circles is the blood glucose - and you see as the insulin production drops, the blood glucose goes up and you make the diagnosis of type 2 diabetes.

But the key problem... there's two key problems: The resistance and the beta cell dysfunction. For this reason people tell you that the beta cells are "burning out", right? And that's why type 2 diabetes is chronic and progressive and eventually, you know, you take medication and you take insulin they take more insulin and more Insulin:

Learned Helplessness

- Fact: Fot most people, type 2 diabetes is a progressive disease
- eventually oral medications may not be enough to keep blood glucose levles normal. Using insulin to get blood glucose levels to a healthy level is a good thing, not a bad one.

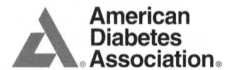

American Diabetes Association®

http://www.diabetes.org/diabetes-basics/myths

And that's the way we tell people to think about type 2 diabetes unfortunately it's not really true.

So the key is to understand what insulin resistance actually is, okay? Where does it come from, how does it develop? In order to understand insulin resistance you got to think about what insulin normally does:

34

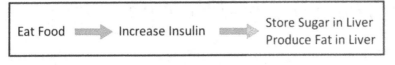

Functions of Insulin:

1. Increase glucose entry into cells
2. Turn on De Novo Lipogenesis

When you eat food insulin goes up, right? Insulin basically tells the body that food is coming in and you should store some of it. So you store sugar in the liver (which is glycogen) and you store fat also. If you eat too much carbohydrate then that is going to be produced by a process called "de novo lipogenesis" into fat. And when you don't eat (which is simply called fasting, that's just a flipside of eating) your insulin falls.

And as it falls, it tells your body to pull some of that sugar and pull some of that fat back out of the system. So as long as you balance your feeding and fasting, you got a well-balanced system, you don't actually gain any weight. Right? Because you eat, you store sugar. You don't eat, you fast, you burn sugar. Right? That's basically all it is.

Insulin does a couple of things: So it lets all this glucose into the cell - but it also produces this new fat. That's the de novo lipogenesis. So there's two functions, not simply one. And this is the way we think about about insulin resistance, it's this lock and key paradigm. That insulin acts like a key on the cell. So this is, for example, a liver cell:

The ‚Lock and Key‘ paradigm

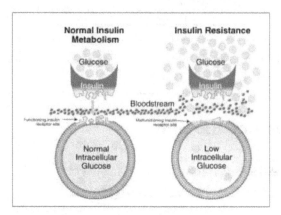

„Internal Starvation" – Cannot drive DNL

You have receptors which is like a lock. When insulin is produced, it opens the gate and it lets all the glucose in. So what we tell people is that insulin resistance is actually a state where this mechanism, this lock and key paradigm, is completely gummed up, okay? So it's not that the lock is defective or the key is defective because you can easily sequence the insulin or the insulin receptor: They're normal.

But something is gumming up the system so all the glucose stays outside and the cell faces this state of "internal starvation", right? So they can't go in.What that means, of course, is that the liver cell cannot produce fat, right? You got no glucose in there, you're not going to produce fat. So what internal starvation looks like is this:

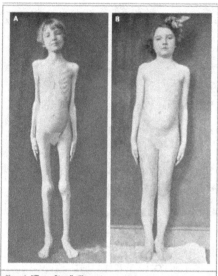

Figure 1. Effects of Insulin Therapy.
These photographs from 1922, in a case described by Geyelin,[11] show a young girl with insulin-deficient diabetes before treatment with insulin (Panel A) and after treatment (Panel B).

Because we know in type 1 diabetes, untreated type 1 diabetes, that the cell faces internal starvation - and you look like the patient on the left. She's starving away you can feed her whatever you want, she can't use it and she basically wastes away until she dies. If you give her insulin, her cells now don't have the internal starvation and she regains the weight - great! We know that's what happens when the glucose can't go in!

But this is what type 2 diabetes looks like:

Internal Starvation?

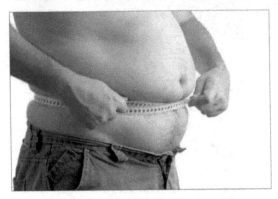

This is what we're calling internal starvation? There's something a little bit wrong with that paradigm of a gummed up lock and key system. There's a paradox here that is not explained by the gummed up lock and key. Because if you look at this liver cell... okay, so insulin pushes the glucose into the cell and if your insulin resistant it doesn't do that. Okay, that's great.

But the other thing this liver cell is supposed to do is turn on production of new fat. So if your insulin resistant you can't produce any new fat. Like that untreated type 1 diabetes you waste away. But that's not the case in type 2 diabetes!

If the glucose is not going into the cell, how is this cell producing tons and tons and tons of fat? Because we know that the type 2 diabetic, the insulin resistant patient, has a lot of insulin resistance has a lot of fatty liver! In fact you always see the fatty liver, right?

So how can this cell... the very same cell, the very same insulin, the very same insulin receptor, be resistant on the one hand to one of the functions - and super-sensitive to the other function? It's not correct! And we have based our entire treatment of type 2 diabetes on an incorrect paradigm!

So what happens in this liver cell, of course, is that you have insulin:

Liver Cells

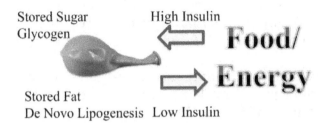

Stored Sugar
Glycogen

High Insulin

⇐ **Food/**
⇒ **Energy**

Stored Fat
De Novo Lipogenesis Low Insulin

Under conditions of high persistent insulin:
Liver becomes full of sugar and fat

As you have insulin, it puts the sugar and the fat into the liver. I've depicted the liver as a balloon, right? So it blows up when you eat. As insulin falls, it comes back out. That's all it is, it's a storage problem. But the problem with fatty liver is that if it fills up with persistent insulin (if you eat a lot of glucose, if you eat a lot of fructose) you're going to fill up this liver cell:

Fatty Liver causes Insulin Resistance

Stored Sugar

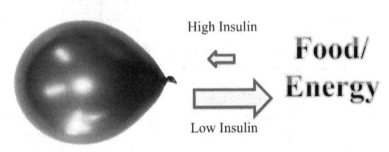

High Insulin

⇐ **Food/**
⇒ **Energy**

Low Insulin

Stored Fat

With insulin acting all the time you're going to keep pushing it into storage. What happens is that you get fatty liver, right? That's not so hard to understand. But it's this fatty liver that's the key to understanding insulin resistance. Because if you have a huge, fatty liver that same dose of insulin is not going to be able to shove any more fat into this fatty liver. And if you don't have insulin then all of this fat and sugar just comes rushing back out, right?

So the reason that you have this central paradox is because this is an overflow paradigm! The glucose can't go into the cell but the fat keeps coming out. If the glucose couldn't go in you couldn't make the fat. But it's not a under-filled cell ,it's an overflowing cell. And this fatty liver precedes the diagnosis of type 2 diabetes. Because it's on that long slow rise where you get the slow rise in the blood glucose, slow rise in the insulin resistance:

Fatty Liver precedes T2D

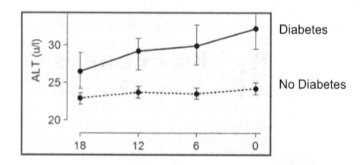

18 months prior to diagnosis of DM
Long ‚silent scream' from the liver

So this is the Whitehall study which shows you the time course of the liver enzymes before the diagnosis of type 2 diabetes. And what you can see is that... they brokaye the group into two groups. One, that eventually developed diabetes and one might eventually didn't. And what was the big difference? Well, if you look at the markers of liver tests you can see that the liver is slowly getting distended and slowly getting inflamed. ALT, which is the marker of liver damage, is slowly going up.

And what they called it is the "long silent scream" from the liver. You can't hear it, you can only see it on the blood test. You might be able to see it on CT or MRI. But it's this big, fatty liver that's the key to understanding the insulin resistance.

So it's really an overflow paradigm, right? The cell is like this luggage:

Insulin Resistance is an Overflow Phenomenon

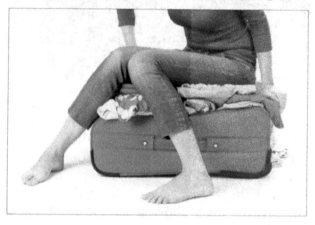

As you fill it up, it's harder and harder to put in more stuff. At first you can put in your clothes fine but those last two t-shirts, you just can't shove them in! So you use more force, you use more insulin you keep shoving stuff in.

But that's not the problem. The problem is not the insulin, the problem is that your cell is overfilled. It's an overflow paradigm. Just like this:

Insulin Resistance is an Overflow Phenomenon

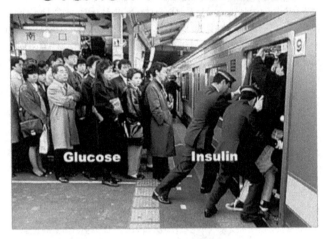

Your cell is like a train, it's got passengers and normally they go in. Insulin opens the door, stuff goes in. Well, what happens if that cell is already filled? If it's already filled with glucose and fat (that liver cell) you keep shoving it in with insulin... that's not the solution. Right? If you have the wrong paradigm!

You think that the Train is not opening the door so you hire these these guys to keep shoving people in. They do this in Japan... But the problem is the glucose stays outside, the passengers can't get in so you keep trying to shove it in. Which is fine at first, then you go to the next stop, you hire more guys, right? You hire more insulin guys keep shoving it in!

And it works for the next stop then you hire more guys to keep shoving it in - until you can't anymore. Then everybody stays outside - you make the diagnosis of type 2 diabetes!

So the key to understanding type 2 diabetes is it's all about the fatty liver:

What causes Fatty liver?

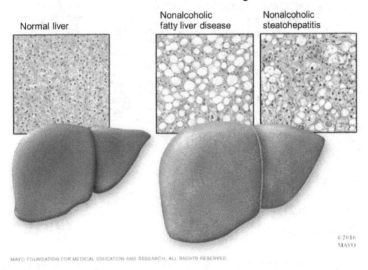

Normal liver | Nonalcoholic fatty liver disease | Nonalcoholic steatohepatitis

©2016 MAYO

The liver cell is just packed with fat so you can't shove anymore in. And that's the whole point! In the meantime, the liver is busy trying to decompress itself off all this fat. So what it does, it's making all this new fat through de novo lipogenesis and it packages out it through triglycerides in the blood.

And it's pouring out this triglycerides and that's why the novo lipogenesis is so high. It's not resistant (remember this is the effect of insulin), it's super sensitive. It keeps trying to push it all out.

So how do you get fatty liver? Well, it's not so hard in geese, right? This is how you make foie gras:

What causes Fatty Liver?

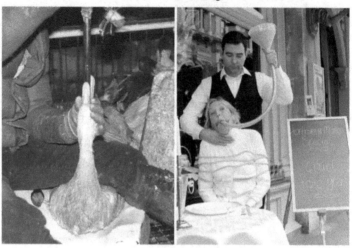

You shove a tube down its neck and what do you feed it? Well, you feed it starch, right? Because you want the liver to make new fat. You don't make new liver fat by eating fat, humans don't do that. The dietary fat does not go to the liver.

But what happens is when you feed it starches - and fructose particularly - you get fatty liver. And that's what happens in humans as well. When you over feed carbohydrates, glucose and fructose, you get fatty liver. And that's how you get insulin resistance:

What causes Fatty liver?
Hormonal Obesity

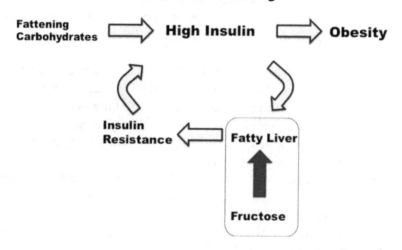

So the key, again, to understanding this is that it's hyperinsulinemia, high insulin. But also this insulin resistance. That's the key to obesity, that's the key to insulin resistance. That's the key to everything. So if you eat a lot of fattening carbohydrates you can stimulate insulin, right? And that will lead to obesity.

But high insulin levels over a long period of time are also going to stimulate fatty liver - as you produce this new fat through de novo lipogenesis which is going to lead to insulin resistance. Which is then going to lead to high insulin levels.

Again: The fructose doesn't do this. This is why everybody used to say "Fructose? Well, it's not that bad, sugar is not that bad for you!" Because fructose does not raise your blood glucose, it's a different sugar altogether. And it doesn't raise your insulin levels. So people say "Oh great, fruit sugar! It's great!" It's not great!

The problem with fructose is the way it's metabolized in the body. It's metabolized solely in the liver. Okay? So if you take sucrose (sugar is sucrose which is equal parts glucose and fructose)... when you eat glucose and fructose you have equal amounts. If you take an average-sized man, 170 pounds, you eat a pound of sugar, you get half a pound of glucose and half a pound of fructose.

The half pound of glucose is metabolized by 170 pounds of the body. So every tissue in your body, every part of your body is going to use that glucose. But none of it uses the fructose, right? So that half a pound of fructose is metabolized by five pounds of liver.

So what does the liver do with it? Well, the liver could turn it into glucose but you alreadygot lots of glucose - so it turns it into fat! So instead of 170 pounds of tissue using glucose... your cells are kind of helping themselves out at this 'all you can eat glucose buffet' - nobody touches the fructose. The fructose goes into the liver and gets turned directly into fat!

So what it means is that if you only have five pounds of liver, the glucose and the fructose are not equally bad for you. The fructose is like 20 times as bad as the glucose! So the starches, the rice and pasta and that stuff, that's all glucose. So the fructose is really where the money is.

So glucose plus fructose is what gives you fatty liver. Which gives you the insulin resistance. And what's glucose and fructose? It's sugar!

Glucose + Fructose =
Fatty Liver =
Insulin Resistance =

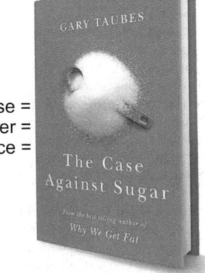

And everybody knows this, right? Every diet says to cut the sugar. Even those diets that say "Oh, you should eat starch. But, by the way, you shouldn't eat sugar as well!" Right? Because the fructose is really the big problem and it's the fatty liver. So that's insulin resistance. It's all about, predominantly, fructose but also glucose and a lot of fatty liver.

What causes this "beta cell burnout"? Doesn't it burn out, doesn't it die out? That's why once you get type 2 diabetes, it's irreversible. Right?

Well, again we know that's not true - because we can prove it! If you look at studies on bariatric surgery... this is a study comparing medical intervention to bariatric surgery:

Surgery cures diabetes

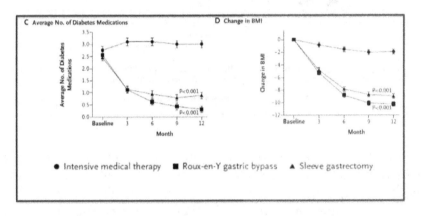

Bariatric Surgery versus Intensive Medical Therapy in Obese Patients with Diabetes
N Engl J Med 2012; 366: 1567-76 Schauer PR

So this is weight loss surgery, they cut your stomach to the size of a walnut and then they rewire your intestines so you can't absorb what you put in your stomach. And what happens of course is that the people on the left started out with almost three diabetic medications. And very quickly, within three months, many of them were off all their medications with normal blood glucose. Their diabetes completely reversed!

And this happens even far before much weight is lost, right? So if you're telling me that the pancreas has burned out... this study tells you that you can take a man or woman with 20, 30 years of type 2 diabetes with 3, 4, 5 medications - and completely reverse it. Completely!

Not just in one person, in everybody! And you can do the same thing with gastric banding. Castric banding is where you put a little... it's essentially a belt that cinches around your stomach so you can't eat. Again, if you look at their weight it goes down:

Gastric Banding cures Diabetes

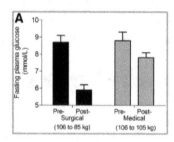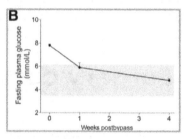

A: Fasting plasma glucose and weight change 2 years after randomization either to gastric banding or to intensive medical therapy for weight loss and glucose control

Adjustable gastric banding and conventional therapy for type 2 diabetes
JAMA 2008; 299: 316-232 Taylor R Dia Care 2013; 36: 1047-1055

American Diabetes Association.

But if you look at the blood glucose: When you start it's 8 which is type 2 diabetes. Within a week it goes down into the normal range, right? Again, before a lot of weight is lost.

So this pancreatic beta-cell that produces the insulin is completely functioning again. It wasn't burned out at all!

And if you compare fasting versus bariatric surgery you can actually get the exact same effect! So here's a comparison where they fasted people using very low calorie diets before and after surgery:

Fasting vs. Bariatric Surgery

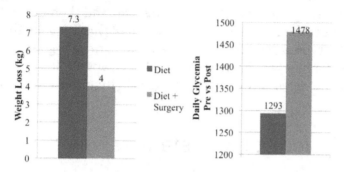

Rapid Improvement of Diabetes After Gastric Bypass Surgery: Is It the Diet or Surgery?
Diabetes Care. 2013 Mar 25, Lingvay I
http://www.ncbi.nlm.nih.gov/pubmed/23530013

The point of the the fasting was they wanted to shrink that liver. Because when they do the surgery, if you have a big, fatty liver it's very hard to get in, hard to work things. So they know that if people don't eat, that liver shrinks right down. When that fatty liver shrinks right down, of course the insulin resistance goes away. Because insulin resistance is from fatty liver!

So you can see from the left hand side: The weight loss, comparing the fasting to the surgery - and the fasting actually causes more weight loss. And if you look at the blood glucose, it gives you lower blood glucose, which is actually better.

If you look at the counter point study:

Decrease in Pancreatic Fat

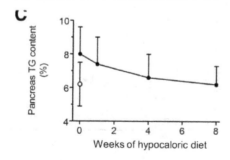

Weeks of hypocaloric diet

Taylor R Dia Care 2013; 36: 1047-1055

49

What you see is that the pancreatic fat slowly goes down. So your body (when it has nothing to eat) is pulling that sugar, pulling that fat preferentially out of the liver and then out of the pancreas. Because it's the fatty infiltration of these organs that is causing the type 2 diabetes. So as the pancreatic fact goes down, the beta cells recover. So they weren't burnt out at all!

This is the restoration of the beta cell function and of the insulin response:

Restoration of Beta Cell Function

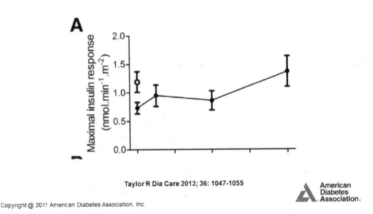

Taylor R Dia Care 2013; 36: 1047-1055

American Diabetes Association.

Restoration of First Phase Insulin Response

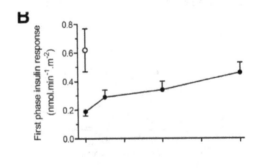

Taylor R Dia Care 2013; 36: 1047-1055

American Diabetes Association.

They were merely clogged with fat! And that's tremendous news because it means that this whole notion, this whole paradigm, that type 2 diabetes is chronic and irreversible is completely untrue. It's a completely reversible disease!

So the idea... the way you need to think about type 2 diabetes is basically like a sugar bowl:

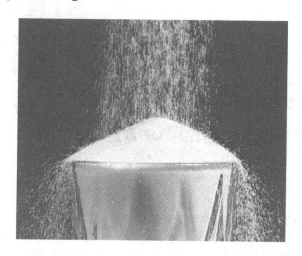

Your body is like a sugar bowl. It can hold a certain amount of sugar. But once it's completely full - as you eat the sugar it just spills out into the blood. Remember sugar, we're talking glucose and fructose. It spills out into the blood. If you have type 2 diabetes somebody says "Well, you have type 2 diabetes now. Let me give you insulin because we think that the sugar can't get into the - so we need to give you insulin!" What does that that insulin do?

Well, it doesn't get rid of the sugar in the blood. What it does is it takes our sugar in your blood and crams it back into your body. Right? And then the next time you eat, that sugar bowl is still full. So you take more insulin and then you cram it back into your body again.

Your body takes it for a while, sends that sugar out into the eyes, into the kidneys. It turns a lot of that into fat - and you haven't fixed the problem. You keep doing this, year after year, you take more insulin or drugs that stimulate insulin. You cram it back into your body. And so what happens after 10, 15, 20 years? Well, your whole body just starts to rot:

The End Game

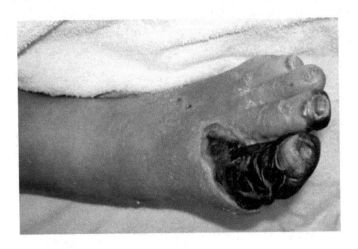

And that's what happens! Your eyes go... you go blind. Your kidneys, you go on dialysis. You have gangrene and diabetic foot ulcers. Every part of your body has too much sugar. That's it, that's it, that's the whole pathophysiology!

And what we've done is we've completely misunderstood the disease. Because normal is this:

Normal	**Insulin Resistance**	

Glucose

Cell

"Internal Starvation" Paradigm

"Overflow" Paradigm

Normal is on the left. You have glucose, you have a cell, you have some glucose inside the cell. So if you think type 2 diabetes about is about internal starvation then the correct response is to give as much insulin as you need to shove back glucose from the outside inside.

But if insulin resistance is really an overflow paradigm then that treatment is completely utterly wrong. Because you're taking that glucose from the outside and cramming it into the cell - which is now overfilled, has way too much glucose inside. And it's desperately trying to pump out this fat!

It's the wrong treatment! And if you give the wrong treatment, guess what? Everybody dies.

You get a huge worldwide epidemic of obesity, of type 2 diabetes, all because you didn't understand it. Right? So if you think about the internal starvation model, we already know it's wrong. We've known it for close to 10 years. Because under this paradigm you can take the insulin shove it into the cell and you will get better.

But the Accord study showed that, yes, you can give people insulin and medications:

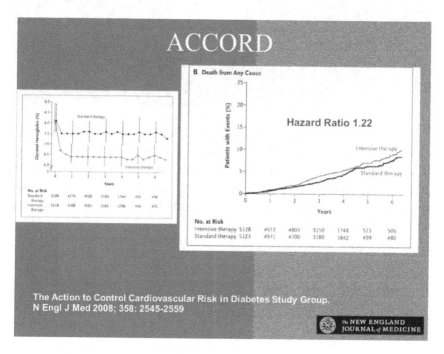

What you see is that you give you more medication your blood glucose goes down. But remember, it doesn't get rid of the sugar in the body, it just crammed it into the cell. And what happens? Well, you die more often - there's a 22% increased risk of death! And everybody says there were problems with this study. But it wasn't this one study it was like 7 or 8 studies.

The Advance study was the same:

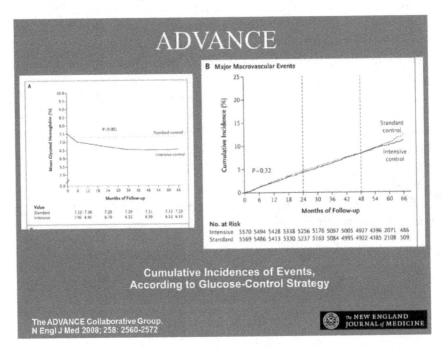

You can give medications to lower the blood glucose but you can't make people healthier, right? And the VADT showed the same thing that TICO studied the eLIXIR study. There's study after study after study. And if you look at all of them what you see is that... when you take all of them together they show you what you already knew:

Meta-analysis of intensive glucose control in T2DM: mortality

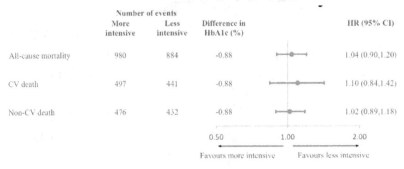

	Number of events More intensive	Number of events Less intensive	Difference in HbA1c (%)		HR (95% CI)
All-cause mortality	980	884	-0.88		1.04 (0.90,1.20)
CV death	497	441	-0.88		1.10 (0.84,1.42)
Non-CV death	476	432	-0.88		1.02 (0.89,1.18)
			0.50	1.00 2.00	
			Favours more intensive	Favours less intensive	

• Meta-analysis of 27,049 participants and 2370 major vascular events from
  - ADVANCE
  - UKPDS
  - ACCORD
  - VADT

HR, hazard ratio; CV, cardiovascular
Turnbull FM et al., Diabetologie 2009; 52: 2288-2298

Which is that taking insulin doesn't make you any healthier.

The good news is that you can actually reverse type 2 diabetes completely naturally! As long as you understand this overflow paradigm. Because there's only two things you need to do: If your body has too much sugar (that's all type 2 diabetes is, your body has too much sugar):

Step one is **Don't put any more in!** It's a low carbohydrate diet. That's why it works so well! That's why study after study after study shows the low carbohydrate diet works to reverse type 2 diabetes. It's not that hard to understand.

So what's the drug equivalent of a low carbohydrate diet. Well, we have a drug that can block the absorption of carbohydrates. It's a drug called Acarbose. So? you take the drug, it blocks the absorption of carbohydrates and the sugar doesn't go into the body. Which is great, right? Because it's a full sugar bowl. You're blocking it, you're not putting it in.

But it doesn't lower the blood glucose very much. And the other thing is that you get all this indigestion and so on, so people don't use this much. But there's a study in 2003, a randomized study three point three years of follow-up:

Lowering glucose *withour raising insulin* improves outcomes

Figure 2. Effect of Acarbose on the Probability of Remaining Free of Cardiovascular Disease

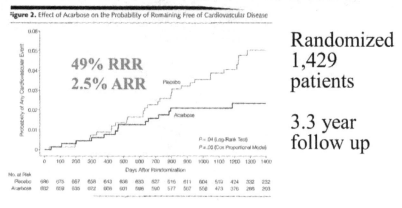

49% RRR
2.5% ARR

Randomized
1,429
patients

3.3 year
follow up

Acarbose Treatment and the Risk of Cardiovascular Disease and Hypertension
in Patients with Impaired Glucose Tolerance
JAMA 2003; 290: 486-494

And what you see is that you can reduce the risk of heart attacks and strokayes - cardiovascular events on the left - by almost 50%! Right? You're not lowering the blood glucose much but you're lowering your heart attack rate by 50%. Because you're not putting sugar in to a situation where you have too much sugar. That's it!

What's step two? Step two is **you'd burn it off!** If you have too much sugar in the blood don't put any more in and get rid of what you have inside. That's it! And that's intermittent fasting.

So again: Do we know it works? Well, of course we know it works. If you don't eat your blood sugar drops, right? We know that. So what's wrong with that? Don't eat blood, sugar drops, don't take your insulin. That's it.

But your body is getting rid of the sugar so that you're actually getting better from your diabetes. And we have a drug equivalent of this as well. So a new class of medications called the SGLT-2s, makes you pee out the sugar, pee the glucose in the blood.

It doesn't lower the blood glucose a lot but this is a recent study, EMPA-REG, and it was published I think last year:

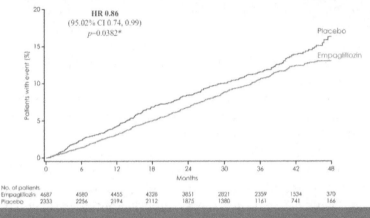

EMPA-REG MACE

HR 0.86
(95.02% CI 0.74, 0.99)
p=0.0382*

Placebo

Empagliflozin

Patients with event (%)

Months

No. of patients									
Empagliflozin	4687	4580	4455	4328	3851	2821	2359	1534	370
Placebo	2333	2256	2194	2112	1875	1380	1161	741	166

*Two-sided tests for superiority were conducted
(statistical significance was indicated if p ≤ 0.0498

What you can see is that this is the risk of cardiovascular events and... what you see with the Empagliflozin is that you can reduce the rate of heart attacks by 15-20 percent! Even though you don't lower the blood glucose. You're getting rid of the sugar in the body - and that's what makes you healthier because that's the whole problem. Right?

So this is a very powerful paradigm! We have to understand that this is not some kind of chronic, irreversible disease. And we tell people this all the time! You have obesity, you're insulin resistant "Well, it's your fault! You ate too much fat, you've didn't exercise enough. You should eat less and move more! It's your fault!" That's what we tell people all the time.

But it wasn't! It was really the failure of the doctors, of the researchers, to understand that type 2 diabetes is not about too much sugar in the blood. It's about too much sugar in our whole body! That's what you need to get rid of. You can't simply take the sugar in your blood and shove it in your body and pretend that you're better.

It's like if you have garbage in your kitchen and instead of throwing it out you throw it under the sink. "Great my kitchen is nice and clean!" And then, when there's more garbage, you throw it into your bathroom, right? "Hey great my kitchen is clean"

Your doctor pads himself on the back, "Oh, your blood glucose is so good, your A1C is so good!" Right? But what's the problem? You haven't thrown out the garbage and your whole house just starts to smell. And then the doctors says: "Well, that's what happens you know. It's chronic, it's irreversible." But it wasn't! We've proved it already, why can't you accept that fact? You just have to know how to treat it!

But again the opportunity before us is enormous - because we have now the possibility that you can actually just completely cure the whole damn disease, right?

And if you think about it, it's an incredible notion. Because if you don't have diabetes, then you don't have diabetic nephropathy (that's kidney disease), you don't have to do dialysis, right? You don't have diabetic foot ulcers, you don't have any blindness from type 2 diabetes.

You don't have heart attacks, you don't have the strokayes, you don't have the cancer. None of that. Right? And it's all available to us! Without any drugs, without any surgery and without any cost!

Can We Cure Type 2 Diabetes?

No Diabetes – no diabetic nephropathy, no diabetic foot ulcers, diabetic retinopathy, reduced stroke, MI, cancers

No Drugs, No Surgery, No Cost

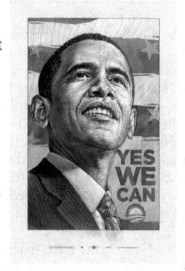

If you don't eat you don't have to pay for food, right? You're saving money! What could be simpler? And you're treating your type 2 diabetes. So this is the whole idea of this conference. That these diseases which cause so much pain, so much suffering - and we've treated them for so long with the wrong paradigm: "Just take your medications".

No, that's not the case. This is a dietary disease, it demands a dietary solution! And that's all, that's all we need. And we can do it! We can do it any time we want to because as long as you have knowledge, you don't need the infrastructure, you don't need the hospitals, you don't need anything.

You don't need any infrastructure, you can do it. In that world... that world, we can see it now! That world that is free of type 2 diabetes and free of all of these heart attacks and strokayes and all of that. It's there! Right?

But it's not up to me! It's up to you, it's up to all of you! To tell your friends, your family "Yes!... tell your doctors. Tell your doctors! And if you are a doctor tell your patients! It's all here for us, it's all here for the taking - we can see it through that open door!

You can see it through that open door and we just have to walk through that threshold. We're inviting you to come walk with us through that threshold to that world... without diabetes without pain, without medication, without insulin. And guess what? That world starts today!!

Thank you!

Time to get started...

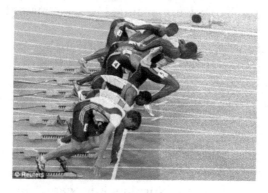

www.intensivedietarymanagement.com

What I've learned: Fasting vs. Eating Less: What's the Difference? (Science of Fasting)

What's the difference between eating less food and eating no food? Well, let's look at two different situations:

In 1944, a study called the Minnesota Starvation Experiment was conducted and was designed to understand the effects of caloric restriction on the body in order to gain some knowledge that would help people starving in the aftermath of World War 2. Thirty-six healthy men with an average height of 178cm (about five foot ten) and average weight of 69.3 kilograms (or 153 pounds) were selected.

For three months, they ate a diet of 3200 calories per day. Then, for six months they ate only 1570 calories. However, caloric intake was adjusted to attempt to have the men lose 1.1 kilograms per week, meaning some men got less than 1000 calories per day.

The foods given were high in carbohydrates, things like potatoes, turnips, bread and macaroni. Meat and dairy products were rarely given.

During the six months, the men experienced profound physical and psychological changes. Everyone complained that they were too cold. One subject talked about having to wear a sweater in July on a sunny day. The subjects' body temperature dropped to an average of 95.8 degrees Fahrenheit (35.4 degrees celsius). Physical endurance dropped by half, and strength showed a 21 percent decrease. The men experienced a complete lack of interest in everything except for food, which they were obsessed with. They were plagued with constant and intense hunger.

There were several cases of neurotic behavior like hoarding cookbooks and utensils. Two participants had to be cut from the experiment because they admitted to stealing and eating several raw turnips and taking scraps of food from garbage cans. At first, the participants were allowed to chew gum, until some of the men began chewing up to 40 packages a day.

Now compare all this to the case of Angus Barbieri, a Scottish man who in 1965 fasted for over 380 days straight. That is he took in no food whatsoever. Nothing but water, black coffee and straight tea for just over a year. He lost 276 pounds, going from

456 pounds to 180. A case report published by the Dundee University Department of Medicine in 1973 said "...the patient remained symptom-free, felt well and walked about normally," and "...prolonged fasting in this patient had no ill-effects."

There were no complaints of mind numbing hunger and he kept the weight off. For several years, his weight stayed around 196 pounds.

This of course is not a perfect comparison: With the case of Angus, there's only one subject and his starting weight was drastically higher compared to those in the Minnesota Experiment. However, it does illustrate some very interesting points about just how different of a physiological response you get from fasting (that is, eating nothing) compared to eating less, or caloric restriction.

Dr. Jason Fung, a Toronto physician specializing in kidney disease, and author of the *Obesity Code,* says that compared to fasting, caloric reduction will result in: less weight loss, more lean mass loss (i.e. more muscle loss), and more hunger.

Let's start by talking about hunger. In Upton Sinclair's 1911 book *The Fasting Cure,* he writes about fasting as a means to improve health.

In describing his first couple attempts at fasting he writes "I was very hungry for the first day. The unwholesome, ravening sort of hunger that all dyspeptics know. I had a little hunger the second morning, and thereafter, to my great astonishment, no hunger whatever. No more interest in food than if I had ever known the taste of it."

Sinclair recommends to do quite long fasts - around 12 days or so. In a section addressing concerns about fasting, he writes "Several people have asked me if it would not be better for them to eat very lightly instead of fasting, or to content themselves with fasts of two or three days at frequent intervals. My reply to that is that I find it very much harder to do that, because all the trouble in the fast occurs during the first two or three days. It is during those days that you are hungry."

Then he says: "Perhaps, it might be a good thing to eat very lightly of fruit, instead of taking an absolute fast. The only trouble is that I cannot do it. Again and again I have tried, but always with the same result: The light meals are just enough to keep me ravenously hungry!" In the bookay he says you will know when you should finish fasting, because your hunger will "return."

He quotes a letter he received from a 72 year old man saying "After fasting 28 days I began to be hungry, and brokaye my fast with a little grape juice, followed the next day with tomatoes, and later with vegetable soup." He quotes several other letters he received from readers and this disappearance and reappearance of hunger is a common theme. Everyone who wrote to him fasted for at least 10 days, saying they only broke their fast when hunger "returned." This phenomenon runs contrary to the idea that one would get hungrier and hungrier as long as they don't eat.

However, most people have experienced for themselves that this is not the case. Some will find that they are not hungry at all in the morning or at least they are not as hungry as they are for lunch or dinner. But unless you are eating in your sleep, the morning is when you have gone the longest without food.

Some of this can be explained by the hormone Ghrelin. Ghrelin, known as the "hunger hormone" has been found to increase appetite and weight gain.

A study at the Medical University of Vienna looked at patients participating in a 33 hour fast. Their ghrelin levels were checked every 20 minutes. interesting is ghrelin is lowest at 9 AM, which is when they have gone the longest without eating. And, ghrelin comes in waves and overall doesn't rise during the period the subjects were fasting. Then, ghrelin rises in sync with normal lunch and dinner times, as if the body had learned to expect food at that time.

However, that ghrelin rise spontaneously decreases after 2 hours without food. I've experienced this kind of spontaneous decrease in hunger myself many times when I was working as a consultant. Lunch time would come and I would be hungry, but I was too busy to eat so I just kept working. Pretty quickly I forgot about eating and wasn't particularly hungry until dinner time.

This is very helpful to keep in mind if you're doing a long fast or even if you're starting intermittent fasting - you're going to get annoying waves of hunger, especially around the times that you usually eat. But, it won't get worse, the hunger will simply go away if you are patient.

Another study concerning ghrelin was done at Aarhus University Hospital in Denmark and it shows what happens if you do a longer fast.

They looked at the ghrelin levels of 36 subjects who fasted for 84 hours. So, did they get increasingly hungrier throughout the fasting period? Well, no. Their ghrelin followed similar rhythms each day but actually decreased the longer they fasted. Going longer without food actually made them less hungry!

This gives credence to what Upton Sinclair and his readers said about hunger disappearing after the first 3 days of fasting. I've done a couple 5 and 6 day fasts in the past myself and this was indeed the case. Actually, I did a day fast last week and, again, the 4th day was when I was the least hungry.

Another thing that may be contributing to this phenomenon is that you are entering ketosis. Ketosis is a physiological state where your metabolism switches to using primarily fat for energy. For this reason ketosis is popular as a weight loss method, but it has many other benefits including better physical and mental efficiency.

Ketosis occurs when you restrict carbohydrates down to 50 grams or less a day and you don't eat too much protein. Everyone's body is a bit different so you might have to eat even less carbohydrate or may have room for more. But the recommended ratio of a ketogenic diet is to get 5% of your calories from carbs, 25% from protein and 75% from good fat.

A simpler way to enter ketosis is: Just don't eat anything for a long enough time. This is one of the major points in the difference between fasting and caloric restriction. The problem with the subjects in the Minnesota Starvation experiment was that they were eating just enough to keep them out ketosis and keep their metabolism primed for burning carbohydrate (glucose), so they couldn't use their body fat for energy. This explains a lot of things like why they were losing their strength and were very sluggish and cold.

It also clears up why Upton Sinclair said fruit or light meals were just enough to keep him ravenously hungry and far weaker than if he had just eaten nothing.

Insulin is necessary for glucose to get into the cell to be used for energy. When you eat carbohydrates, the pancreas secretes insulin to deal with it and too much insulin hampers the action of something called hormone sensitive lipase which is necessary to mobilize fat and use it for fuel.

Though, keep in mind that grains or refined carbohydrates will provoke a much higher insulin response than, say, green vegetables. Now because the body is having a hard time using its fat for fuel, it will do a couple things: One, it will simply slow down metabolism to preserve energy.

In the Minnesota Starvation experiment, the subjects metabolism dropped by 40 percent. Their bodies didn't have access to its stored energy, and their restricted calorie diets didn't provide much fuel so there's no choice but to slow down the metabolism.

Ironically, in the case of fasting - as Jason Fung points out - metabolism actually goes up. "If you don't do anything about your insulin and just reduce your calories, your metabolism goes down. But what happens during fasting? Well, here's a study of consecutive days of fasting. What happens to your REE - the resting energy expenditure. It doesn't go down, it goes up. You're burning more energy than you did before!"

The other thing the body will do when it can't use fat for fuel is break down muscle into glucose through a process called gluconeogenesis. The body doesn't want do this too much because it's not very smart to completely eat through something as important as muscle. But when it can't access its own stored energy, it's more likely to resort to this. This is why you'll experience more muscle loss on caloric restriction than if you ate nothing.

When you are fasting, Human Growth Hormone is released. As the name implies, Human Growth Hormone is an anabolic hormone - a hormone conducive to growth.

In Leningher's Principles of Biochemistry textbook, they give the example of how injecting the human growth hormone gene into a mouse makes it unusually large. As explained in Guyton's Textbookay of Medical Physiology: "Growth hormone also mobilizes large quantities of free fatty acids from the adipose tissue and these in turn are used to supply most of the energy for the body cells, thus acting as a potent protein sparer."

That is, human growth hormone is protecting your muscles from breaking down. The study I referred to earlier about subjects undergoing an 84 hour fast shows that growth hormone rises significantly after the second day of fasting.

As mentioned earlier, you should enter ketosis sometime within the first 3 days or so of fasting, and it depends on how much you are moving around and what your diet was like before starting the fast.

The state of ketosis is a great indicator that your body is making good use of its stored body fat for energy. In Tim Ferriss' book *Tools of Titans*, Tim talks about his first clinically supervised 7 day fast. For some sort of liability reasons, he wasn't allowed to exercise or leave the facility. Considering exercise is a potent stimulator of human growth hormone and will deplete glucose stores, not getting any exercise is a great way to prevent yourself from getting into ketosis during a fast.

It's also a great way to lose muscle. Tim says he lost 12 pounds of muscle during the overly restrictive clinically supervised 7 day fast. But, when following a protocol designed to get him into ketosis as soon as possible (involving things like 4 hours of brisk walking) he did a ten day fast and apparently lost zero muscle mass.

One last factor in ketosis preserving muscle is leucine. When you're in ketosis you have a higher fasting blood leucine level. And leucine is a key branch chain amino acid that has an anabolic effect on the body so it preserves lean body mass. A lot of people interested in building muscle may be worried that fasting or a ketogenic diet wouldn't work for them because insulin and therefore carbohydrates are necessary for protein synthesis (i.e. muscle growth). But actually leucine fills that role and is a good trigger for protein synthesis.

So, just to sum all this up:
compared to a conventional calorie restricted diet, fasting means
- you lose more weight in the form of fat
- you keep more muscle
- you have more energy, and
- you are less hungry

If proper weight loss is your goal, it might be better to eat nothing at all rather than eating a conventional low calorie diet.

Studies cited
(in chronological order)

Chapter 1:

Metabolic slowing with massive weight loss despite preservation of fat-free mass.
Johannsen DL et al., J *Clin Endocrinol Metab.*, 2012; 97(7); 2489-96

Metabolic Adaptation Following Massive Weight Loss (..)
Knuth ND et al, *Obesity* 2014; 22: 2563-2569

Long-term changes in energy expenditure and body composition after massive weight loss (...)
Krupa Das S et al, *Am J Clin Nu* 2003 78: 22-30

Comparative Physiology of Fasting, Starvation and Food Limitation, Autor: Dr. Kevin Hall, NIH

Resting energy expenditure in short-term starvation is increased as a result of an increase in serum norepinephrine.
Zauner C et al, *Am J Clin Nutr* 2000; 71(6):1511-5

Alternate-day fasting in nonobese subjects: effects on body weight, body composition, and energy metabolism.
Heilbronn LK et al, *Am J Clin Nutr* 2005; 81:69-73

Starvation – in 'Transaction of the American Clinical and Climatological Association'.
Cahill, G. 1983; 02/1983; 94; 1-21

Improvements in Coronary Heart Disease Risk Indicators by Alternate-Day Fasting(..)
Bhutani S et al, *Obesity* (2010) 18, 2152-2159.

Influence of Fasting and Refeeding on Body Composition.
Drenick EJ et al, *Am J Public Health Nations.* 1968; 58 (3): 477-484

Chapter 2:

Whitehall II study.
Lancet 2009; 373: 2215-2221

Surgical treatment of obesity and ist effect on diabetes: 10-y follow-up
Am J Clin Nutr 1992: 55 (Suppl.): 582S-585S

Bariatric Surgery versus Intensive Medical Therapy in Obese Patients with Diabetes
N Engl J Med 2012; 366: 1567-76 Schauer PR

Adjustable gastric banding and conventional therapy for type 2 diabetes
JAMA 2008; 299: 316-232

Type 2 diabetes: etiology and reversibility
Taylor R Dia Care 2013; 36: 1047-1055

Rapid Improvement of Diabetes After Gastric Bypass Surgery: Is It the Diet or Surgery?
Diabetes Care. 2013 Mar 25, Lingvay I

The Action to Control Cardiovascular Risk in Diabetes Study Group.
N Engl J Med 2008; 358: 2545-2559

The ADVANCE Collaborative Group.
N Engl J Med 2008; 258: 2560-2572

Intensive glucose control and macrovascular outcomes in type 2 diabetes
Turnbull FM et al., *Diabetologie* 2009; 52: 2288-2298

Acarbose Treatment and the Risk of Cardiovascular Disease and Hypertension in Patients with Impaired Glucose Tolerance
JAMA 2003; 290: 486-494

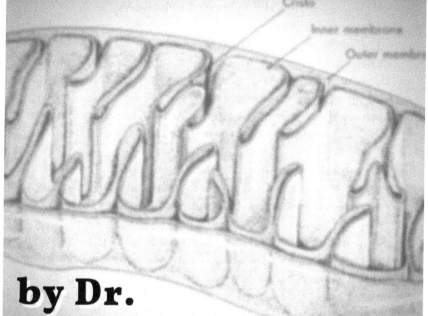

SUMMARY OF:
CANCER AS A METABOLIC DISEASE

by Dr. Thomas Seyfried

ON THE ORIGIN, MANAGEMENT, AND PREVENTION OF CANCER

25% of the royalties of this book will be donated to Dr. Seyfrieds research!

This research will actually make a REAL impact, as it studies the real causes and treatment opportunities of cancer!

This book is a summary of Dr. Thomas Seyfrieds book "Cancer as a metabolic disease" and comprises transcripts of his talks and interviews, as well as texts by his collegue Dr. Dominic D'Agostiono and Travis Christofferson (whose foundation will be supported by this book).

Here the original Book description:

The book addresses controversies related to the origins of cancer and provides solutions to cancer management and prevention. It expands upon Otto Warburg's well-known theory that all cancer is a disease of energy metabolism. However, Warburg did not link his theory to the "hallmarks of cancer" and thus his theory was discredited.

This book aims to provide evidence, through case studies, that cancer is primarily a metabolic disease requring metabolic solutions for its management and prevention.

Support for this position is derived from critical assessment of current cancer theories. Brain cancer case studies are presented as a proof of principle for metabolic solutions to disease management, but similarities are drawn to other types of cancer, including breast and colon, due to the same cellular mutations that they demonstrate.

Sources

Chapter

1) Text (editors revised transcription) and slides based on Youtube video:

Channel: „ Low Carb Down Under "

Channel-Url:

https://www.youtube.com/channel/UCcTTiHZtNpiqD2EubIO5HFw

Title: " Therapeutic Fasting - Solving the Two-Compartment Problem "

Video-Url: https://www.youtube.com/watch?v=tIuj-oMN-Fk

2) Text (editors revised transcription) and slides based on Youtube video:

Channel: „ Low Carb Down Under "

Channel-Url:

https://www.youtube.com/channel/UCcTTiHZtNpiqD2EubIO5HFw

Title: " Dr. Jason Fung - 'A New Paradigm of Insulin Resistance' "

Video-Url: https://www.youtube.com/watch?v=eUiSCEBGxXk

3) Text (editors revised transcription) based on Youtube video:

Channel: „ What I've Learned "

Channel-Url:

https://www.youtube.com/channel/UCqYPhGiB9tkShZorfgcL2lA

Title: " Fasting vs. Eating Less: What's the Difference? (Science of Fasting) "

Video-Url: https://www.youtube.com/watch?v=APZCfmgzoSo

Thanks to Dr.Jason Fung for his important work to cure people of our modern diseases!

His website: https://thefastingmethod.com/
(formerly intensivedietarymanagement)

His YouTube Channel:

https://www.youtube.com/channel/UCoyL4iGArWn5HuoV_sAhK2w

———————————

Version 1.01   24. August 2020

———————————

CPSIA information can be obtained
at www.ICGtesting.com
Printed in the USA
BVHW091145150621
609530BV00013B/2756